Your Dry
Are

The Ultimate Guide To
#NoMoreDryHair

Heather Katsonga-Woodward

www.NenoNatural.com

BY THE SAME AUTHOR

To Become an Investment Banker:

Girl Banker®'s Bullet Point Guide to Highflying Success

Chichewa 101 - Learn Chichewa

in 101 Bite-sized Lessons

Black Girl - Getting to Wealthy:

Build Super Savings

Black Girl - Getting to Wealthy:

Build a Booming Business

The SECRET Rules of Money

Neno Natural's DIY Hair Products Series

Foreword

For years there have been misconceptions on how to care for natural hair as well as its true beauty and essence.

I am a "Natural Hair Enthusiast" and have been an advocate of natural hair since 2010. Even though I stopped relaxing in December of 2008 and big chopped in October of 2009, I had to lead by example and show others the transformation natural hair can have on your mind, body and spirit.

I suffer from alopecia and started noticing balding and thinning around my edges when I was 26.

As a young woman, this had a major impact on my self-esteem. I had issues with my hair falling out when I styled and washed it because it's the most fragile type, 'type 4' in addition to being very fine. It needs to be handled with supreme care.

I turned to the internet for help on how to save my

hair and even spent countless hours and money visiting dermatologists. It turned out that all I needed was a basic understanding of how to care for my hair and the best practices for developing a regimen (with the proper products) that was right for me.

Since natural hair is on the rise, it is becoming more popular on television, in magazines and on the internet.

As naturalistas learn to celebrate and appreciate the beauty of their kinky, coily or curly textures, the creativity of styling options and hair care options is growing abundantly.

Issues pertaining to hair growth, dryness, shedding and so on can be understood with the information provided within this book. This book provides solutions for overcoming these obstacles and other major hair difficulties that naturals encounter.

With basic tips on how to manage your mane, you can begin to understand what your hair needs to thrive and be healthy hair. Those who are entertaining the idea of starting a natural hair journey or those who are currently on a natural hair journey will find this an easy read.

Remember that everyone will have a different experience when it comes to their hair journey. Be patient with your hair and do not be afraid to switch up your regimen or products if you see your current practice is not working. Do not compare your hair to others who have "gone natural", "returned natural" or "big chopped" around the same time that you did.

It's the ups and downs of being on a natural hair journey that add to the joys and experience you have. Have a healthy, happy hair journey!

Ngozi

Ngozi Ali, Vlogger, youtube.com/nalia1908

Publisher's Note

Every reasonable effort has been made to ensure that the information presented in this guide is accurate at the time of going to press. No responsibility for loss or damage occasioned to any person acting, or refraining from action, as a result of the material in this publication can be accepted by the editor, the publisher or the author. No part of this publication may be reproduced in any manner without prior written consent from the author.

First published in Great Britain & the United States in 2015 by Zumex Press.

www.NenoNatural.com

youtube.com/hkatsonga

ISBN 978-1-909184-21-3

For #LittleZeusy,

My bff for life.

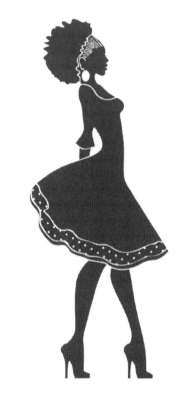

About The Author

Heather Katsonga-Woodward is the founder of the natural hair blog NenoNatural.com. She designs hair care products and blogs about kinky and curly hair; her specialty is resolving dry hair issues. Heather's goal is to help women enjoy managing their hair whatever their hair goals are.

Neno Natural grew to over 400,000 Facebook fans, and 40,000 email subscribers in under two years. Building on this success, in 2014 Heather launched a coaching program supporting others to build a 6-figure product business called "*The Money Spot™.*"

In a previous life, Heather was an investment banker at Goldman Sachs and HSBC. She resigned from the banking industry in 2012 to pursue her business interests full-time and to enjoy a more flexible lifestyle.

Heather lives in London with her husband, Harry and their son, Chester (also known as Little Zeusy on social media). She maintains a hair & life vlog at youtube.com/hkatsonga – check it out to meet her and her family.

Key Resources For You

NenoNatural.com has lots of free information on hair; use the search bar to look for specific topics or browse the list of categories at NenoNatural.com/hair-blog.

For hair profiles from fellow naturals go to: NenoNatural.com/queens.

Or download the Queen of Kinks magazine on iPhone, iPad or Android.

If you'd like to make your own hair care products go to: NenoNatural.com/courses.

For my hair and life vlog with my husband, Harry, and my son, Little Zeusy: YouTube.com/hkatsonga.

For 10% off your order of the *Queen of Kinks* boxed set of products for dry hair, use the coupon code SOFTH4IR on amazon.com or SOFTHAIR on amazon.co.uk and at NenoNatural.com. Quick links are at NenoNatural.com/queenofkinks.

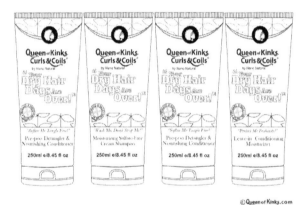

Table of Contents

Introduction

This book is designed to be a fast read. Nobody's got time for waffle. The book has one aim: to help you grow longer and healthier hair by avoiding dryness.

Excessively dry hair breaks much more easily than hair rich with moisture. Kinky and curly hair is naturally more prone to dryness than straight hair. But if you can avoid the dry hair problem you will soon be enjoying kinks, curls and coils that look and feel healthy.

This book was inspired by my own experience. In March 2011 I encountered severe hair breakage for no apparent reason. I got scared and stopped relaxing my hair, a ritual, that like many others, I had been practicing since I was four years old. It was time to transition to natural hair. Within 18 months I could tie all my hair back and most importantly, it was healthy.

After my transition, dryness plagued me for a long time. It made hair management a lot less fun. Once I mastered how to prevent dry hair I actually started to enjoy the maintenance of my natural kinks! This guide will cover the best of what I've learned about good hair management. This includes the use of high quality products and as the founder of one of the best lines for dry hair, *Queen of Kinks, Curls & Coils* (Queen of Kinks in brief), I'll be introducing you to this amazing brand too.

Chapter 1: The Hair Rule

Since I started managing natural hair in early 2011 I have learnt that there is only one rule:

YOU are the
QUEEN of **YOUR**
KINKS, CURLS & COILS

Consider any tips you hear from others as mere suggestions; if you try them and they don't work for you, ditch them and try something else!

Sometimes two people will appear to have the same type of hair but their hair will react completely differently to the same product. For instance, some hair types remain curly even after the application of a relaxer whereas other hair types become bone-straight.

Before Relaxer

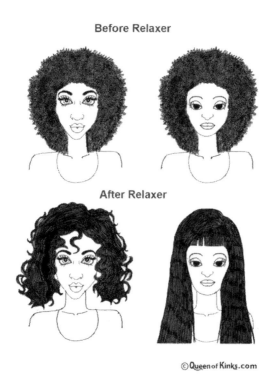

After Relaxer

© Queen of Kinks.com

Chapter 2: Hair Types

Natural hair comes in four main "types": 1, 2, 3 and 4. These types can have subsets categorized from a to c with increasing tightness or density of curls.

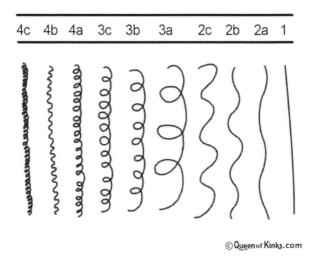

©QueenofKinks.com

- **Type 1** is completely straight hair
  - o It has no subsets
- **Type 2** hair is wavy.
  - o It has three subsets: 2a, 2b and 2c
- **Type 3** hair is loosely curled

- o It has three subsets: 3a, 3b and 3c
- **Type 4** hair is the curliest type of hair.
  - o It has three subsets: 4a, 4b and 4c.
  - o 4c is the curliest type of hair with curls so tight they are coily or kinky.

Hair type in itself is not the most important thing. What matters is that hair type determines how hair should be handled.

Curly hair has a greater tendency for dryness and the curlier it is, the drier it tends to be. This is because the oil naturally produced by hair, sebum, has trouble making its ways down the kinks and curls to moisturize the tips.

All Type 4 hair is very kinky/curly/coily but type 4C (the most kinky), is the driest and most vulnerable to breakage; it needs to be treated with reverence.

The terms kinky, curly and coily are frequently used interchangeably but there are subtle differences: coils are small, compact curls; they look like a small spring. In the strictest sense kinky hair is hair that has a zigzag pattern as opposed to a clear curl or coil. I'll refer to kinkies, curlies and coilies collectively as kinky-curlies.

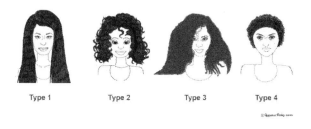

Type 1   Type 2   Type 3   Type 4

Because coils and kinks tend to be so compact, coily and kinky hair tends to be much longer than it appears.

Kinky, curly and coily hair elongates when wet and shrinks back to a tighter kink, curl or coil as it dries; this is referred to as shrinkage.

Chapter 3: Growth Potential

On average, hair grows 0.5 inches per month. You can expect 3 to 5 inches of hair growth a year after trims. Harsh treatments like straightening, excessive braiding and the use of hair chemicals will cause some breakage and result in even less retention of hair length.

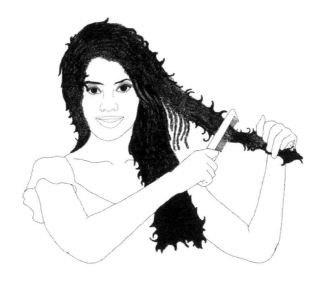

© Queen of Kinks.com

Kinky, curly and coily hair is slightly more

prone to breakage than straight hair because the bonds in hair are weaker at the "bend" points.

If you have very kinky hair, treat it with great care.

Chapter 4: Maximum Hair Growth

Hair does not continue growing forever.

The growth cycle can be as short as 1 year and as long as 10 years. On average it is 4 to 7 years, this limit is genetic and cannot be changed.

If your hair growth rate is 4 inches per year and your genetic limit is 5 years, the maximum length you can achieve is 20 inches of hair before trims.

If you have fast hair growth of, say, 6 inches per year but your genetic cycle is only one year, your hair will not grow beyond 6 inches. It may be less if you trim it to keep ends neat.

What is *your* maximum length? It's not an exact science especially as hair growth is influenced by factors such as diet, exercise, smoking and so on and these behaviours can change over time.

One way to get an idea is to take regular length checks and also to keep track of approximately how much hair you trim off so that you can add this back on to the estimate of your hair growth rate. Over a 12-month period look at your records for an idea of how fast your hair grows.

If you take regular length checks over say, 3 years, you will have a more accurate idea of how fast your hair grows.

Those who opt to shave all their hair off in a "Big Chop" are better able to keep track of length because, by definition, they start at zero on "Big Chop" day.

Managing your hair well, taking vitamins and using high quality hair products will only allow you to reach your genetic limit *not* to exceed it.

That said, hair never stops growing; different hairs on your head are at different stages in the growth cycle. This is why you don't go completely bald at certain points in your life.

About 90% of the hairs on your head are in their growth phase *(Anagen)*.

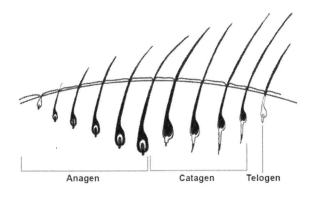

©QueenofKinks.com

When a hair reaches the end of its growth

cycle it stops growing and detaches itself from the blood supply (*catagen*); it then rests (*telogen*) and finally it sheds (*exogen*) and a new hair takes its place.

Shedding is a natural and unavoidable process and up to 100 hairs on your head shed daily.

These hairs either fall out independently or are pulled out during styling. If you have braids or dreadlocks the hairs due to shed don't fall out because they are restricted from doing so.

In the chapters that follow I provide a set of tips to help you reach your maximum potential hair length.

Good hair growth is made of two elements:

1. Treating your hair well

2. Using good quality products.

Beautiful hair is mostly the result of great hair management. Using high quality products will support your efforts but only if your hair is cared for regularly.

Chapter 5: Detangling

Detangling is the one crucial stage of natural hair management that is not required when you have relaxed (or straight) hair.

Why Detangle?

Well-detangled hair is:

- Less likely to break when you're washing and conditioning it
- Less likely to break when you are styling and handling it
- Easier to comb, style and manage

Video: How To Detangle & Prevent Tangling of Natural Hair

DETANGLING TIP 1: Only detangle damp hair

Hair that is either too dry or too wet is more

likely to break than damp hair.

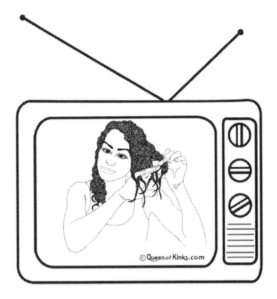

DETANGLING TIP 2: Plasticize hair before you detangle it

Plasticizing is softening hair by using a bit of water and a good quality detangler such as *Queen of Kinks* '*Soften Me, Tangle Free!*' *Pre-poo Detangler.*

If you don't have a detangler, detangle using a

rinse-off conditioner (not a leave-in conditioner) if you are about to wash your hair or use a leave-in moisturizer/conditioner if you are just styling your hair for the day.

DETANGLING TIP 3: Finger-detangle first

Fingers are more adept at detangling than combs. They can work their way through complex tangles more easily without breaking your hair.

DETANGLING TIP 4: Mainly use wide-tooth combs (if you move on to using combs at all)

They are much more gentle on hair.

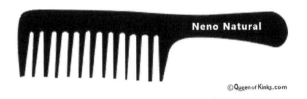

If your hair has been thoroughly detangled with fingers first, then a wide-tooth comb, it will more readily accept a comb or brush with finer teeth.

Some kinky-curly-coilies don't use combs at all and strictly finger comb their hair. This practice doesn't work for everybody.

Chapter 6: Wash & Condition

Handling your hair during the wash and condition process is an opportunity for hair tangling and breakage.

WASH TIP 1: One shampoo a week is adequate

Dry hair does not need to be washed as often as most other types of hair; it is not necessary. Excessive washing will draw out already scarce moisture and increase the likelihood of breakage.

WASH TIP 2: Use a gentle, sulfate-free shampoo

Most shampoos use sulfates as the cleaning agent or "surfactant". Sulfates are commonly used because they are a lot cheaper than other surfactants and they are very strong so product makers only need to use a small quantity to get the desired effect – they blitz every oil out of your hair, even the good oils that hair needs to retain moisture.

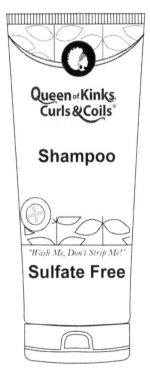

The majority of buying consumers have greasy hair so the hair industry focuses on satisfying their hair need. However, for dry hair, sulfates are too strong a cleaning agent; they wash out too many of the good oils leaving hair too dry.

WASH TIP 3: Co-wash if you need to wash your hair more than once a week

If you feel like you need a more regular wash (for example, if you exercise heavily), add one or two extra washes a week using only conditioner and no shampoo (this is called a co-wash).

Queen of Kinks '*Wash Me, Don't Strip!*' *Moisturizing Sulfate-Free Shampoo* is sulfate-free. *Queen of Kinks* '*Soften Me Tangle Free!*' *Conditioner* can be used to co-wash hair.

Wash & Condition Frequency

Whilst a weekly wash is adequate for most, some kinky-curlies wash their hair more or less frequently than this without any negative consequences. Experiment with the frequency of your hair washes to see what works best for you.

WASH TIP 4: Avoid the squeaky clean feeling!

You know that squeaky clean feel you normally get when you wash your hair with a regular shampoo? That is what you are trying to avoid if you have dry hair.

Squeaky-clean means you've stripped the hair of a lot of it's moisture and natural oils. That's good for greasier hair types but not so good for dry hair.

Washing hair with conditioner (co-washing) does not strip hair as much as using shampoo does, and is therefore less damaging. That said, conditioner is not a cleanser, it's designed to stick good stuff onto your hair. If you repeatedly co-wash without ever shampooing you're applying the good stuff in conditioner to dirty, oily hair.

If, in between your weekly shampoos you sweat a little bit only, your hair won't need an extra wash. If you feel dirty however, you might want to wash it just to feel clean and this is when co-washing comes in handy.

More than three washes a week is excessive for most dry-haired folk. But some people co-wash almost daily and don't find it detrimental because they always moisturize their hair properly afterwards.

A weekly shampoo is critical because some ingredients in conditioner, e.g. oils, butters and some silicones, are designed to be washed off with shampoo.

Silicones have many benefits for hair so rather than avoiding them altogether, learn which ones best suit your hair type and regimen.

The ins and outs of silicones is beyond the scope of this book but I do have a comprehensive blog on the topic at NenoNatural.com, search:
What Are The Best Silicones For People On A Co-Wash Regimen?

Washing Hair & Length

The frequency of your hair washes should change with the length of your hair.

WASH TIP 5: The longer your hair gets the less often you need to wash it

Short hair is more welcoming (and forgiving) of regular washes as it doesn't tangle so easily.

Tangling

Long hair is more likely to get tangled during

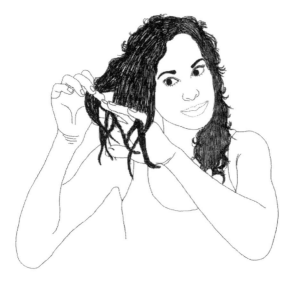

© QueenofKinks.com

your wash session; the process of detangling it, though essential, provides yet another opportunity for breakage.

Infuriating tangles aren't only a problem for kinky and curly hair types; they can also be a big problem for people with very long, straight hair. Regardless of the curl pattern, or lack thereof, the longer your hair gets the more cumbersome handling it becomes.

Grease & Dirt

Fortunately, it takes more time for long curly hair to get greasy and dirty, in general. If you wear it up in protective styles, rather than down and loose, it doesn't need to be washed as often. This is because the sebum produced in your scalp has a longer distance to travel. If your hair is kinky, curly or coily, its journey to your hair tips is all the more difficult and takes more time. Therefore the longer your hair is, the drier its tips will be.

The tips of your hair are the oldest section of hair so the cuticle will have, over time, been eroded away through styling and washes; hair tips therefore need more moisture.

Wash & Go

It would be great if we could all just wash, condition and hit the road but for many kinky-curlies this is a recipe for disaster.

WASH TIP 6: Wash & Gos work best on

- Short hair
- Straight or loosely curled hair

Once type 4 hair grows beyond the shoulders, attempting a Wash & Go can leave you in tears because:

1. The tangling and matting is indescribable!
   You'll wake up with your hair hugging your scalp like a carpet and lifting it off to stretch and detangle will take longer than you probably have on a working day.

2. The shrinkage is exhausting – it makes styling extremely challenging.

3. You will inevitably have more breakage than you would during a normal wash.

Some 3c naturals also cut out Wash & Gos after a certain length because it can make hair much harder to manage for the same reasons above.

Chapter 7: Chemicals to Avoid

The products you use on your hair matter.

Certain chemicals dry hair out; make it more likely to break; clog up the pores on your scalp or simply do more harm than good to your hair.

Good quality hair products can be costly. Whilst it can seem that cheaper alternatives work exactly the same way, keep in mind that the damage inflicted upon your hair by the low quality ingredients found in cheap products, can take ages to reveal itself.

It took me ages to see that my hair was getting thinner and thinner; luckily I noticed before it was too late to save my hair from irreversible thinness due to damaged hair follicles. To avoid finding yourself in the same situation, I suggest the following:

PRODUCT TIP 1: Read product labels; know which chemicals are best avoided

If you have dry hair and want to retain optimal length you should consider avoiding products that contain any of the following:

1. Gluten
2. PABA or DEA (paraaminobenzoic acid and Diethanolamine)
3. Parabens – parabens are not bad for hair in themselves but have been linked to cancer
4. Paraffin
5. Petrolatum and mineral oils
   Because petrolatum is very cheap, a lot of hair products targeted towards low budget consumers have traditionally contained a lot of petrolatum (e.g. Blue Magic, Sulfur 8 etc.)

Petrolatum coats hair in a heavy film that makes subsequent efforts to moisturize your hair futile; it is also hard to wash off with a gentle, sulfate-free shampoo.

6. Phthalates
7. Propylene Glycol
8. Sulfates: sodium or ammonium laureth or lauryl sulfate (SLS/ALS)

Note: I used to have silicones on this list but after carrying out extensive research and learning the differences between various types of silicones I removed them from the list. Some silicones are good for hair; they are water soluble and more proficient at detangling hair than any other ingredient.

I explain the good vs. the bad silicones in a series of blogs at: nenonatural.com/hair-blog/category/silicones

PRODUCT TIP 2: Ingredients are listed in descending order of their quantity

The lower on the ingredients list a chemical is, the lower its concentration is within that product.

According to *The Science of Black Hair* by Audrey Davis-Sivasothy, as a rule of thumb, if you see any ingredient placed sixth or lower on an ingredients label there likely isn't enough of it in there to cause you concern.

For instance, I noted that Cantu Shea Butter has petrolatum listed as the 7th or 8th ingredient but I find it still works reasonably well for moisturizing my kinks and curls.

PRODUCT TIP 3: Where possible go for products made by natural hair companies

In 2013 mainstream hair brands targeted at non-Caucasian people jumped onto the natural hair opportunity.

I tried many of these so-called "new" products, some made by popular, long-standing brands, and I was normally left disappointed; they were not that new at all if you looked at the ingredients list. Most had little change to the content of their existing product lines and were just rebranded to appeal to people with natural hair.

Companies use simple marketing tricks such as headlining "new" products with descriptions that evoke very natural or nourishing imagery like 'banana-infused' or 'coconut-based.'

On the other hand, niche companies that specialize in natural kinky and curly hair have grown from the desire to tackle the needs of natural hair specifically: dryness, lack of moisture and curl definition.

These products genuinely cater to the needs of hair that has not been chemically treated and as a consequence, you are a lot more likely to be satisfied with the results they produce.

Finally, note that even though natural hair brands are generally better, make sure you check their content like any other as they too can be misleading.

PRODUCT TIP 4: Don't fall for brands' marketing gimmicks

Read the label. You will find that some products marketed as being "natural" contain harsh chemicals so it's always best to check the ingredients before paying.

I have in the past regretted paying A LOT of money for brands targeting kinky and curly hair without reading the label only to find that they contain too many ingredients that I like to avoid. And more importantly, they didn't work well on my hair at all.

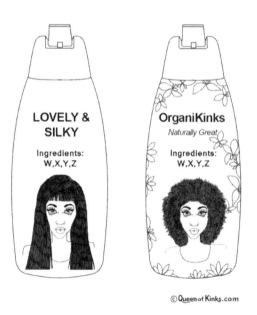

© QueenofKinks.com

To illustrate the point, these two products are

identical but they have been branded differently to appeal to different types of consumers. This is exactly what happens in the world of hair products.

Note: a name like OrganiKinks will make some think the product line is organic even though the product makes no such claims. Branding experts know this and use words in a specific way to imply something that may not be true. Indeed a tag line like "naturally great" will make some people think the product contains only natural ingredients even if it does not.

It doesn't necessarily make the product bad for you, it just means don't assume things are what they seem.

Caveat emptor ~ buyer beware!

Chapter 8: Moisturizing Dry Hair

Water is your friend, dry-haired girl!

MOISTURE TIP 1: Spritz with water regularly

Kinky/curly hair is very vulnerable to dryness; it can lose a lot of moisture even over the course of one day. The number one moisturizer for natural hair is water.

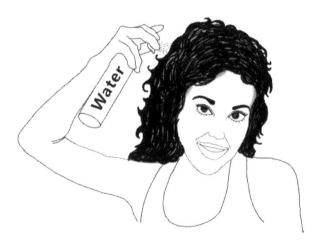

© Queen of Kinks.com

Water will soften hair and keep it hydrated so that it is less prone to breakage and more likely to retain length.

Spritz your hair using a spray bottle at least twice daily: in the morning and in the evening.

Relaxed and heat-straightened hair doesn't like water so if you're moving from relaxed back to natural this is a bit of a revelation. You can officially jump into a pool without thinking: *I can't wet my hair*.

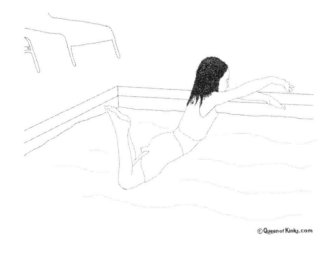

© QueenofKinks.com

MOISTURE TIP 2: Spraying your hair with water regularly cannot replace your weekly wash and condition.

Spraying water into your hair helps to hydrate it for the day or night but after 7 to 10 days you should give it a proper detangle, wash and condition to hydrate it thoroughly.

When you drench your hair fully in water any bits you miss when you spritz it also get hydrated.

Personally, I noticed that whenever I spritzed my hair the edges were getting neglected. That doesn't happen when I wash my hair properly.

MOISTURE TIP 3: Deep condition weekly.

Is your conditioner a deep conditioner? If not

then you definitely want a deep conditioner for dry hair.

There are 5 main types of conditioner:

Instant conditioners are designed for daily use – they are surface acting only, that is, they don't penetrate through your hair cuticle;

Cream-rinse conditioners are good for detangling and heat protection;

Deep conditioners boost moisture, protein and softness. They also strengthen hair by working their way into the cuticle to hydrate and strengthen from within the hair fiber;

Moisturizing conditioners reduce frizz, boost moisture and hair elasticity;

Protein conditioners temporarily rebuild damage along the hair's cuticle.

Some people purchase multiples types of conditioner for different functions but you can get away with owning just a deep conditioner. It is strong enough to work beneath the cuticle thoroughly moisturizing your hair and doesn't contain too many protein ingredients to risk over-proteinating hair.

I specifically mention over-proteinating because many naturals worry about adding too much protein to their hair; indeed, hair that has not been chemically altered doesn't need much protein. Relaxed hair needs many more proteins to replace those lost during the straightening process.

MOISTURE TIP 4: Do NOT deep condition more than once a week

Given the benefits of deep conditioning you'd

be forgiven for thinking that the more you do it, the better, right? – *Nuh-uh*, it doesn't work like that.

If you deep condition too regularly you might incur breakage from excessive moisture.

Some kinky-curlies take moisturizing a little too far and "baggy" their hair in a shower cap too often, wash and condition far too regularly and in come cases even sleep with conditioner in their hair. I'll take a moment here to tell you that this is completely unnecessary; there is no conditioner out there that needs more than half an hour (max) to do its work. One lady who wrote to me only learnt this lesson after waking up with a bald patch on her head; I kid you not.

Excessive moisture is bad because it can lead

to a weaker protein structure in hair. Your hair becomes more porous so the moisture you add escapes too quickly. The result is hair that breaks easily because it is too dry, weak, limp and too stretchy.

If you want to wash your hair more often, for instance, because you exercise frequently, don't let your deep conditioner sit every time: apply and rinse off within 5 minutes to avoid breakage from too much moisture.

Alternatively, get a more watery instant or cream-rinse conditioner to use in between deep conditions.

If it says "suitable for daily use" or something along those lines, it's very mild and okay for more regular use; it is not a deep conditioner. This type of conditioner will tend to be quite watery.

MOISTURE TIP 5: Understand the pH of products

Ideally you should try to use a shampoo and conditioner within the same product line or test the pH of your chosen products to ensure they complement each other

Conditioner is meant to be more acidic than shampoo. The lower pH of the final product used in the hair cleansing process (typically the conditioner) helps to seal off the hair such that the hair cuticles are smoothed down properly. Flattened cuticles are less subject to damage and hold moisture in better.

A shampoo and conditioner within the same product line will be developed with this feature in mind.

For example, the shampoo of one brand may have a pH of 4.5 and the conditioner 3.8 so that your hair is properly sealed off.

But if you then go and use a conditioner of another product line whose pH is 5.0 (designed to work with a shampoo of pH 5.6), this sealing off process won't happen correctly. This is why it helps to stick to the same line of hair products.

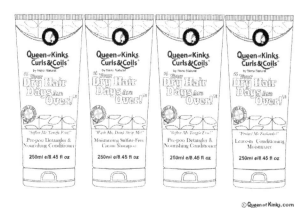

© QueenofKinks.com

MOISTURE TIP 6: Finish every wash off with a cold rinse

Washing your hair with warm water helps to dislodge dirt and oil. Warm water also increases your hair's porosity i.e. the cuticles open up so that all the good stuff from your shampoo and conditioner is easily absorbed.

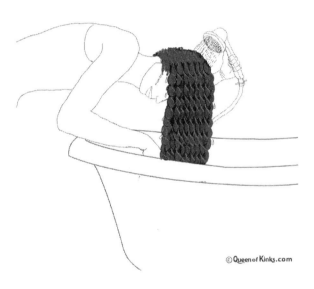

© QueenofKinks.com

Rinsing your hair in cold water at the end of the washing process will help to flatten the hair cuticles again and lock in all that moisture.

I also do this when I wash my face. It helped to clear up my acne.

So, wash with warm water and rinse your final conditioner off with cold water – it does not have to be freezing cold, just as cold as you can stand.

MOISTURE TIP 7: Opt for pure, natural oils and butters for hair use

In addition to water the following natural oils and butters are easy to find and are documented as having great benefits for hair. The list below is by no means exhaustive:

- Argan oil
- Avocado oil
- Castor oil
- Coconut oil or butter
- Grapeseed oil

- Jojoba oil

- Olive oil

- Shea butter

- Sunflower oil

- Sweet almond oil

If you want more details on different oils and butters including how they benefit hair, get a copy of the following two books:

- **DIY Hot Oil Treatments Course (Book 1, DIY Hair Products): How to Blend Carrier Oils & Essential Oils for Great Hair (Neno Natural's DIY Hair Products)**

- **DIY Hair Butters Course (Book 2, DIY Hair Products): A Primer on How to Make Whipped Hair & Body Butters (Neno Natural's DIY Hair Products)**

These two books detail even more great oils and butters for hair than listed above.

Search "Neno Natural's DIY Hair Products" on Amazon for the full series of 6 books.

The kinkier, curlier or coilier your hair is, the more benefit you will find from oils and butters.

If your hair strands are fine or generally quite silky you may find oils and even more so, butters, too heavy for you. In this case you wouldn't use them for sealing your hair, you would only use them for hot oil treatments.

MOISTURE TIP 8: Apply moisturizer to your hair before any oil

Repeat this to yourself a few times: "oil is not a moisturizer."

Oils and butters help to lock in moisture, however, they are NOT moisturizers themselves. You should only apply them onto hair that has already been hydrated and moisturized with a water-based product.

Oil and water do not mix, so oil, if used at all, must be applied last so that it locks-in moisture and stops it from escaping.

Oil is fantastic at locking-in moisture. Two common moisturizing methods:

- In the LOC method, a water-based moisturizer (**L**iquid) is applied first, then **O**il, then a more buttery or **C**reamy moisturizer.

- In the LCO method, a water-based moisturizer (**L**iquid) is applied first, then a more buttery or **C**reamy moisturizer, then **O**il.

MOISTURE TIP 9: A good, moisturizing cream can keep your hair soft for 3 to 5 days without re-application if you just

add water daily.

If you twist your hair using a cream moisturizer, when you untwist the plaits all you need to do is spritz your hair with water and fluff it out to 'reactivate' the cream. In the video, *No more dry hair: how to keep natural hair moisturised for 4 days* (youtube.com/watch?v=TrjjdYh69FI), I show how to do this on type 4 hair.

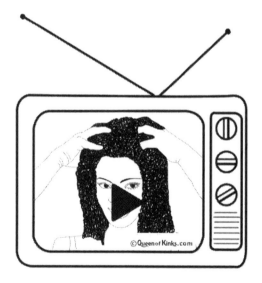

My hair is mostly 4c with some 4b curls at the front and back. And even with such tightly curled hair, sometimes a quick spritz with water is all it takes to soften and reactivate the moisturizer and soften my dry hair.

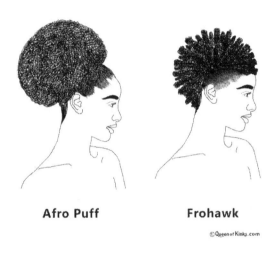

Afro Puff   **Frohawk**

©QueenofKinks.com

Importantly, you can make hair management easier by embracing shrinkage; just style your hair in shrinkage-friendly styles such as afro puffs and frohawks as it shrinks between washes.

Chapter 9: Stimulating Hair Growth

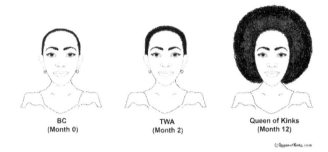

BC
(Month 0)

TWA
(Month 2)

Queen of Kinks
(Month 12)

© QueenofKinks.com

GROWTH TIP 1: Use essential oils to maximize hair growth

Essential oils are highly potent, naturally derived oils that are documented as having active properties. Some essential oils are well known for cleansing hair, some promote hair growth and others help with maintaining healthy looking hair.

The most popular and well-documented hair beneficent essential oils are:

- Cedarwood

- Lavender
- Rosemary
- Thyme
- Ylang Ylang

Neno Natural's Hair Growth Stimulator includes all of these great essential oils except for ylang ylang.

It's perfectly fine to make your own oil blends, however, if you wish to do this, use essential oils with extreme caution as direct skin contact with undiluted essential oil can result in burns or an allergic reaction.

You don't need to use a lot because essential oils are very potent; a few drops of oil is plenty. Specifically, for every 30ml (1 ounce) you only need 10 to 12 drops.

GROWTH TIP 2: Massage your scalp regularly

Massaging the scalp encourages blood to flow to it. Blood brings with it all the nutrients needed for hair growth and health.

Neno Natural's Hair Growth Stimulator can be applied directly to hair because the essential oils sit in a base of jojoba and grapeseed oil; it can be used as a conditioner, for scalp massage or for hot oil treatments. It is available on Amazon at and nenonatural.com and periodically on eBay.

Chapter 10: Heat and Hair

If it were up to your hair, it would avoid heat completely. Unfortunately, we don't live in that world so we need tips on using heat without damaging our hair.

HEAT TIP 1: Use heat cautiously

It's a well-known fact that heat frequently dries out and damages hair. – Many people in the natural hair community apply heat to their hair with extreme caution.

The ones that I follow most fervently (i.e. those with the healthiest and or longest hair) claim to almost never use heat.

When I started out, I didn't know heat was 'bad.' It hadn't occurred to me that heat might be one of the reasons that my hair was breaking so badly. I used to blow dry my hair at least weekly as standard, after my wash and condition routine. I stopped doing so after a few months and soon stopped feeling like I needed to blow dry my hair to stretch it.

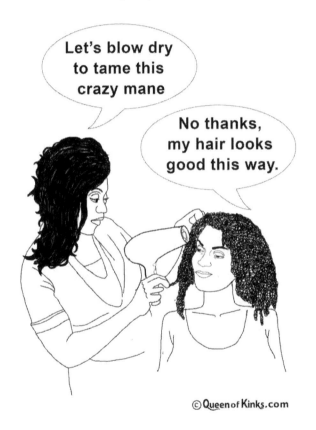

Blow drying is not essential for drying

hair: your hair will dry well and with a great curl pattern if you simply plait or twist it using a good moisturizer (and oil) after you've conditioned it.

Hair straighteners are even less necessary: some kinky-curlies flat iron their hair as a 'treat' once or twice a year but doing so much more than that and it could increase breakage. Those with very fine hair should not risk doing it even that infrequently; people with more coarse hair can get away with using straighteners more frequently.

Now, I only blow dry when I am braiding my hair, currently that's about four times a year.

HEAT TIP 2: Go completely heat free for a few months! No blow dryers and no straighteners.

Because I was nursing my hair from extreme breakage when I first decided to go natural, I decided to completely stop using heat for a while.

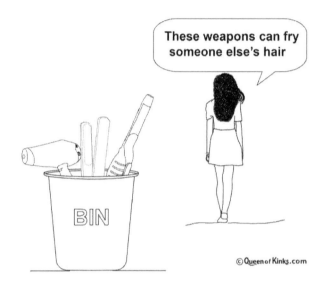

From July 2011 to January 2013, I applied heat only once – on my wedding day, 11/11/11. Once you stop using heat you get used to it and learn how to manage your hair without it.

Heat Safety Tips

HEAT TIP 3: If you must apply heat, do it in the safest way possible:

1. **Wash and deep condition hair** no earlier than the day before you blow dry. Ideally just prior to the blow dry. Don't blow dry dirty hair.
2. **Thoroughly detangle** your hair before you blow dry.
3. **Dry your hair using a microfiber towel** so that it's not too wet and doesn't frizz. Don't rub and scrunch the hair, just tie the microfiber towel over your head and it will soak up the water.
4. **Apply a heat protector**. Coconut oil is an effective heat protector as well as a moisture sealant.
5. **Section hair**. This allows you to deal with any tangles you meet systematically and more easily.
6. **Blow dry using a medium to low heat**. Do not use high heat it could damage your hair.

7. **Blow dry *down* the hair** so that the airflow is in the same direction in which the cuticle layers lie.

8. **Leave a little moisture in the hair.** Bone-dry hair is brittle hair; avoid this level of dryness to prevent breakage.

9. **Finish** the blow dry **with a cold blast of air**. Hot air opens up the cuticle layer and cold hair closes it up sealing the hair, boosting shine and reducing frizz.

If you've become very dependent on heat this might be challenging to start off with but you'll quickly get the hang of managing your hair without using heat.

Chapter 11: Food & Nutrition

FOOD TIP 1: Eat healthily to grow high quality hair

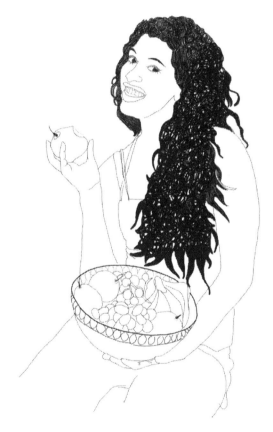

©QueenofKinks.com

When it comes to having healthy hair, nourishment has to come from the inside out. An unhealthy diet equals poor quality hair in the long run.

Hair is low on your body's list of priorities; nutrition goes to the vital organs first and if there's none left for hair and nails, then they don't get any vitamins and minerals. Consequently your hair and nails will crack, break and grow very slowly.

Foods that are rich in protein, iron, vitamin A and B-vitamins are needed for high quality hair.

Changing from a bad diet to a good one won't change the quality of the hair that you can already see, it's your new growth that will look and feel healthier.

FOOD TIP 2: Use a nutrition supplement especially in winter

Can nutrition supplements help? If you have a poor diet and take supplements to substitute for eating well, your hair is still likely to suffer. However, supplements are helpful in making up for any small deficiencies.

For instance, iron deficiency is the most common nutritional deficiency in the world and is especially common in women. Taking an iron supplement will help to make up any shortfall.

I sometimes take a 'skin, hair & nail' supplement for this reason: just in case my diet is low in something. If you're pregnant and taking pregnancy vitamins they will do the job too, don't double up with other vitamins. If in doubt, ask your doctor.

FOOD TIP 3: Eat more of the following fruit and vegetables for healthier hair.

- Apricots
- Bell peppers
- Broccoli
- Carrots
- Cauliflower
- Citrus fruits
- Dark green leafy vegetables
- Mango
- Papaya
- Raisins
- Tomatoes
- Watermelon

FOOD TIP 4: Eat more of the following other foods for healthier hair. *Woman*

cannot live on fruit and veg alone.

- Beans, especially red kidney beans
- Beef
- Bran
- Cheese
- Chicken
- Eggs, especially the yolk
- Fish
- Lentils
- Milk
- Rice
- Soybean

There is no substitute for good quality food. If you eat a lot of junk food and your hair still looks great, it doesn't mean this trend will carry on forever. You can usually get away with looking great on a bad diet when you're young but as you get older your hair (and body) will 'start to complain.'

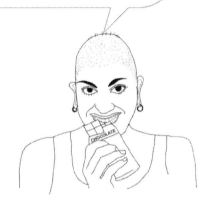

©QueenofKinks.com

Chapter 12: Handling Hair – Combing and Styling

We've been raised to believe that combing and brushing hair is a necessary part of an organized person's life; otherwise hair looks unkempt. Well, I'm here to tell you that this is a myth; some hair types can get away with hardly ever using combs or hair brushes and still look well put together.

Those that are not familiar with natural afro hair may react negatively to afros and big hair in general. Some think it's messy and unprofessional, however, these negative stereotypes are rapidly dissipating and many now accept that there is nothing wrong with hair in its natural state. If you trim your ends, moisturize and finger comb as needed your hair will look healthy and cared for.

This is especially true if you usually put your hair up in protective styles. That said, combs are great for detangling sessions and styling.

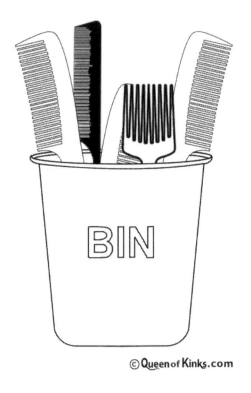

© QueenofKinks.com

I am not against combs and brushes at all, however, they are not your only option. You can easily use your fingers instead of combs.

If you're going to use combs and brushes keep the next few tips in mind.

HANDLING TIP 1: Dry Hair HATES Combs! Don't comb dry hair.

Combing dry hair will increase the rate of breakage. Dry hair is brittle and prone to snapping so it's best to moisturize hair before you comb it.

For the least amount of breakage only comb hair after you have either:

- applied a detangling conditioner such as *Queen of Kinks'* Pre-poo Detangler or;

- plasticized it with water and a hair moisturizer such as *Queen of Kinks'* Leave-in Moisturizer.

HANDLING TIP 2: Use a wide-tooth comb

The best type of comb to use is a wide-tooth comb. Wide-tooth combs have large gaps between each tooth and well-rounded tips so they are less likely to snag hair and are much gentler on thick and kinky-curly hair types.

Some kinky-curlies find that the Denman brush also works well for detangling curly hair types. To make it even better suited for use on kinky and curly hair some people remove every other row on the brush.

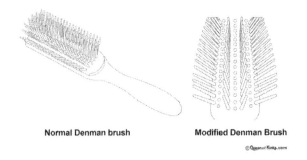

Normal Denman brush   Modified Denman Brush

©QueenofKinks.com

HANDLING TIP 3: Detangle your hair fully before going to a salon

If you go to a hair salon to style or braid your hair etc., they might insist on using a fine-tooth comb. I always say no, however, if you are likely to agree make sure your hair is well prepped for the event by:

1. Ensuring your hair has been deep-conditioned beforehand to soften it and make it easier to comb.
2. Finger detangling well.
3. Using a wide-tooth comb to fully detangle hair strands before using a fine-tooth comb. This way the fine-tooth comb does the least damage possible.

You may find that you need to change salons because some places are better able to handle natural hair than others.

There are definitely some great stylists for

natural hair out there so ask friends for recommendations and read reviews before deciding where to go.

Chapter 13: Sleep & Hair

Hair needs to be shown some TLC before you hit the hay. This is especially true for kinky and curly hair than it is for straight hair.

SLEEP TIP 1: Protect your hair with silk or satin when you go to bed.

There are two things you can do for your hair when you're sleeping:

1. Protect hair from breakage
2. Protect hair from getting matted flat against your head

Dehydrated hair is much more prone to breakage and matting.

Cotton materials are not great for hair because they:

- Draw already-scarce moisture out of your hair;

- Have a rougher texture than silk and satin, so when you toss and turn you create opportunities for breakage.

A satin head cap or a satin pillowcase offers the best protection during sleep because it's slippery and hair just slides along it.

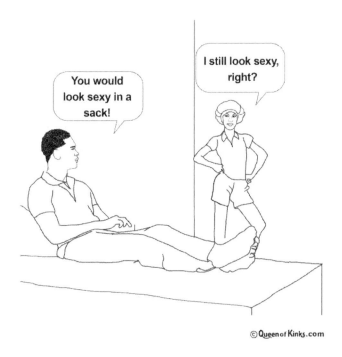

> You would look sexy in a sack!

> I still look sexy, right?

© QueenofKinks.com

You don't need both a satin cap *and* a satin

pillowcase, one or the other is fine.

You'll notice that the hair on top of your head tends to grow faster than in any other place, the fact that it remains relatively untouched during sleep helps with that.

SLEEP TIP 2: Protect hair from getting matted during sleep by twisting or plaiting it.

Sleeping without twisting your hair can cause the strands to stick together and the coils to tighten up, this is matted hair. It's a key problem for type 4 hair.

Matted hair is harder to detangle and style. Twisting your hair before bed may seem like a chore but it saves you a lot of detangling time in the morning. As with all things, once you get into the routine of plaiting or twisting your hair before bed you stop thinking of it as a chore.

If your hair does get matted, spritz it with water and use your fingers to lift the hair out of its matted state. Apply a moisturizer like *Queen of Kinks* *'Protect Me Jealously!'* *Moisturizer* for extra slipperiness and ease of detangling.

Combing matted dry hair without the help of water and a moisturizer will lead to unnecessary breakage.

Chapter 14: Weather

Bad weather can damage hair and dry it out.

Bad weather includes:

- Wind

- Cold

- Extremely air conditioned environments e.g. on flights

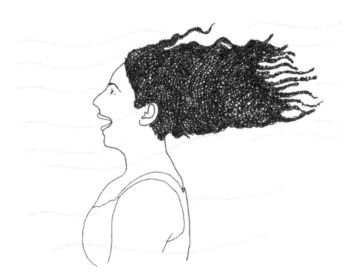

Windy days

© Queen of Kinks.com

WEATHER TIP 1: Ensure your hair is

seldom exposed to bad weather

During winter wear hats and head scarves when you are outside. This is the single best thing you can do for your hair during cold months.

When you are on a long-haul flight take a hat or even better, your satin night hat, onto the plane with you.

Sleeping with your satin hat on will protect your hair in the same way it does when you sleep on a pillow.

To avoid awkward looks on the plane, wear a beanie or other hat on top of the satin cap – no one has to know it's there!

Chapter 15: Hair Styles for Length

Some hairstyles are more conducive to retaining length and preventing dryness than others.

STYLE TIP 1: Wear protective hairstyles to prevent breakage and to hold moisture in for longer especially when the weather is bad.

Hair strands are least protected when they are loose. Part of the reason people with dreadlocks grow such long hair is because it's always packed together; breakage is reduced significantly when the hair strands are together. Also, shed hairs remain matted to the locked strand whereas shed hair falls out when your hair is 'free'.

Protective styles are hairstyles that involve pulling your hair up so the tips are hidden (normally) and the hair does not rub against clothing.

It's obviously more fun to wear your hair out and show it off. But if you wear more protective styles, your hair will thank you with better length retention. Importantly, if you live in a very hot area you will find that your hair is much less dry and brittle at the end of each day.

Protective styles are great all year round but are most helpful when the weather is bad, i.e. very hot, very cold, windy or rainy.

Chapter 16: Braiding

First things first, is it okay to braid your hair? Does it increase hair loss and breakage?

Some people with natural hair prefer not to braid their hair at all, ever. However, braids do not have to be damaging to hair. They can protect or ruin your hair; it all depends on the type of braids you go for.

One of the main advantages of braiding hair is that it gives your hair a rest from combing and handling.

BRAID TIP 1: If time is scarce, braid your hair.

If you're super-busy or pregnant you may be too tired for hair management for prolonged periods of time; braiding provides a useful break from all that daily hair handling. As a new mum I still struggle for time so it's a relief to plait my hair and forget about it for a while.

Braiding To Grow Hair

Here are a few tips for braiding your hair in such a way that you don't get breakage:

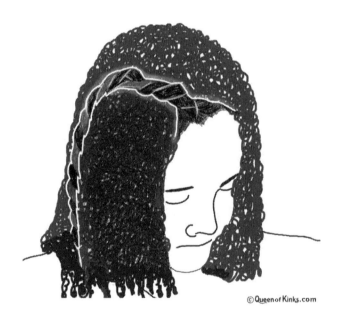

© QueenofKinks.com

BRAID TIP 2: Avoid thin or heavy braids.

Make sure you don't put a relatively large hair extension on a small patch of hair. The pulling impact from the weight of the extension could lead to breakage or worse, pull hair out from the roots.

BRAID TIP 3: Go extension free.

Plait your hair without using extensions, e.g. by doing corn rows or single plaits and twists with your own hair only.

BRAID TIP 4: Do not neglect your hair when it's in braids.

Treat your hair just as well in braids as you usually do. This means deep conditioning, washing and moisturizing every 7 to 10 days.

BRAID TIP 5: Cornrow the front edge.

If you do use extensions, consider cornrowing the hair on the front edge. The edge tends to be more prone to breakage so extra weight from braids can make things worse.

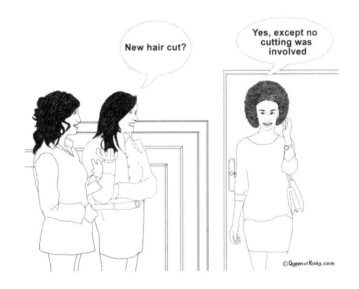

BRAID TIP 6: Water still matters when you're in braids.

Continue to spritz hair with water a few times

a week. This will ensure that when you unbraid the hair it's not dry and brittle.

BRAID TIP 7: Have braid-free weeks.

Don't go from one set of braids straight into a new set; have a break of at least 2 weeks between braids to analyze the state of your hair.

Chapter 17: Frizz Control

The following tips have the double benefit of reducing frizziness in addition to helping to keep dry hair soft.

FRIZZ CONTROL TIP 1: Don't forget to rinse with cold water

Warm water causes hair to frizz a little as the cuticles open up. However, in order to loosen dirt and oils from the scalp and hair during a wash, you need warm water.

To quell frizziness, rinse conditioner out with cool water. This tames frizziness, boosts shininess AND locks in moisture by flattening the hair cuticle.

FRIZZ CONTROL TIP 2: Leave some of your rinse-out conditioner in your hair

According to *The Science of Black Hair* by Audrey Davis Sivasothy, *"If hair dryness and frizziness are major problems after shampooing and conditioning your hair, consider allowing a small amount of your "rinse-out" conditioner to remain in the hair after rinsing for additional control and sleekness."*

I can't vouch for all conditioners but leaving a little product in is certainly something you can do with the *Queen of Kinks Conditioner*. In addition most instant, daily use conditioners are suitable for leaving in.

FRIZZ CONTROL TIP 3: Use a microfiber towel to dry your wet hair

A regular terry towel (made from cotton or a polycotton mix) ruffles up hair fibers and causes the hair cuticle to lift and frizz. Microfiber is much more absorbent than cotton; it soaks up water without you having to rub the towel in your hair.

See **nenonatural.com/hair-blog/category/microfiber** for more on microfiber towels.

FRIZZ CONTROL TIP 4: Try Argan oil

Argan oil is reputed as being the best oil for reducing frizz.

FRIZZ CONTROL TIP 5: Master your hair drying technique

Don't rub or ruffle your hair dry, just tie your microfiber towel around your head and let the water drip into the towel; you can also use a cotton shirt for this. Remember I recommended that you shouldn't sleep directly on cotton pillowcases because cotton soaks the moisture out of hair? Well, in this case we actually want the water soaked out so a cotton shirt is perfect.

Alternatively, if you partitioned your hair using twists or plaits to wash it, squeeze gently down your partitions.

FRIZZ CONTROL TIP 6: Mix gel and moisturizer

For more defined, frizz-free curls, mix a little gel with your hair moisturizer and scrunch (don't rub) this mixture down your hair by lightly squeezing.

Gel, as always, helps to set the style and the moisturizer will smooth the hair down thereby blocking atmospheric moisture from frizzing your hair.

FRIZZ CONTROL TIP 7: Don't keep touching your hair

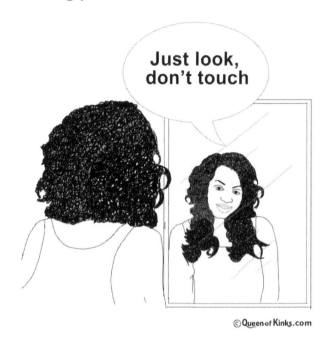

If you keep touching your hair you'll encourage it to frizz.

Lots of touching and rubbing causes frizziness because you tamper with the hair's cuticle layer.

FRIZZ CONTROL TIP 8: Give the ends a little more TLC

Finally, the ends of your hair are older, weaker and therefore more prone to frizz. They need more moisture and are less likely to develop split ends if they're not rubbing against clothing.

Chapter 18: Trimming

TRIM TIP 1: Keep your ends trimmed

Trimming is important because:

1. It helps your hair appear well looked after
2. It smartens up your appearance. Untrimmed hair ends do not look good on any hair type – straight or curly
3. It gets rid of already dry, damaged hair and stops split ends from causing further damage.

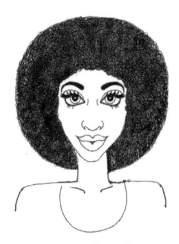

©QueenofKinks.com

Heather Katsonga-Woodward

Damaged hair and split ends are more likely to get tangled with healthy hair than other healthy hair strands; this extra friction encourages more hair damage and increased breakage.

How Often Should You Trim?

There is no hard and fast rule for when you should trim. I would trim:

1. To respond to your hair's needs

You can tell your ends need a trim when they start to look worn out, dry and frizzy. If you don't get rid of those ends they will end up breaking on their own and may also tangle and damage your healthy hair strands.

2. To keep it neat

If your hair is uneven and if you feel it could do with some tidying up give it a trim.

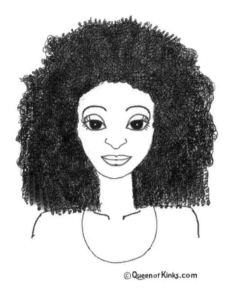

© QueenofKinks.com

3. To stop the ends from getting damaged

"Dust" the ends regularly so that you don't need to trim often. "Dusting" involves trimming so little hair that it looks like dust. This technique helps to stop split ends from forming.

You can dust every 6 to 8 weeks; just snip off a tiny, inconsequential amount.

How To Trim Natural Hair

There are two methods I recommend for trimming hair. Whichever you choose always trim your hair on a wash day using very sharp scissors.

Method 1: Kinkier Hair Types

After you have rinsed out both shampoo and conditioner, apply your leave-in conditioner or moisturizer.

Using a wide-tooth comb make sure your hair is well detangled before you twist it for air-drying.

Twist your whole head. Once twisted trim the end of each twist.

Will your hair be even? It will be even enough.

For more information and a visual of how this works, watch my video tutorial on "How To Trim Natural Hair" at nenonatural.com/hair-blog/how-to-trim-natural-hair.

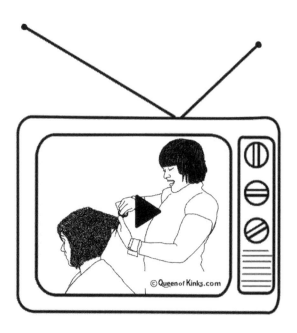

Method 2: Straight Hair & Loose Curls

If, when you pull your hair straight down it reaches below your shoulders, you can do away with twisting it into sections before trimming the ends.

After detangling your hair, comb it down as you would if you were to wear it loosely. Then have someone else trim it for you so that it looks even.

This is the method normally used for straight, wavy and loosely curled hair. It can also work for type 4 after a certain length.

Chapter 19: Building A Regimen

A daily and weekly routine can help to keep your hair soft, healthy and easy to manage.

REGIMEN TIP 1: Maintain a weekly hair routine

Wash Day Routine (Weekly)

This regimen is based on when my 4c/4b hair was medium length. You can copy it or adjust it to suit your own hair and lifestyle.

STEP 1. Finger detangle damp hair...

...because it is far easier to detangle hair when it is just a little damp rather than when it is completely drenched or very dry. Dampen hair and softening it with a detangler such as *Queen of Kinks* '*Soften Me, Tangle Free!*' *Pre-*

poo Detangler; as mentioned before, this is called plasticizing hair.

If you can't get hold of a decent detangler, use a little rinse-out conditioner to detangle.

Short hair detangles more quickly and easily; long hair needs you to allocate at least an hour, sometimes two hours just to detangling. You will have to make time for this process, it can't be rushed. This is why most people leave hair washing for the weekend when they have more spare time.

STEP 2. Shampoo

I only shampoo once a week regardless of how dirty my hair is because I don't want to strip it too much of its natural oils.

I did not section my hair at all when my hair

was short or medium length. The "natural hair gurus" had me believing this is a MUST but I didn't seem to suffer for it.

STEP 2. Shampoo continued...

When my length went a couple of inches past the shoulders I did start seeing the benefit of sectioning. Leaving it loose exacerbated tangles. That was until I started using the *Queen of Kinks 'Wash Me, Don't Strip Me!' Sulfate-free Shampoo*. I started using the product as soon as I formulated it (about a year before it came to market). The creamy nature of this shampoo offers extra slipperiness for detangling, compared to gel textured shampoos.

This means you can get away with leaving hair unsectioned until the very end. See what I mean in the video, *How To Revive Dry Natural Hair From A Matted Mess - No Breakage,* (youtube.com/watch?v=GK3zt_40iHg).

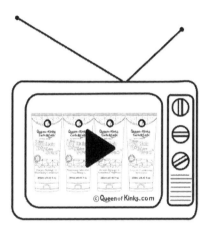

If my hair is already twisted up and I think it's extra dirty, I loosen one section at a time to wash it more thoroughly, re-twist, then move to the next section.

STEP 3. Deep condition, section hair

and twist each section

I used to leave my hair loose during most of the wash process when it was medium length. As it grew longer I started conditioning section-by-section and retwisting each section after conditioning.

I then cover my head in a shower cap, blow dry over the surface, and cover my head in a towel, a thick head wrap or a beanie to trap the heat and deep condition.

With just the shower cap over my head I get on with bathing and rinse my hair once that is done.

STEP 4. Rinse out conditioner and dry hair with a microfiber towel

STEP 5. Moisturize and plait or twist each section.

As you moisturize your hair you might want to use a wide-tooth comb rather than just your fingers to detangle each section a little more.

Apply *Queen of Kinks* '*Protect Me Jealously!*' Leave-in Conditioning Moisturizer to the hair and seal with an oil, such as coconut oil, or with a hair butter.

To minimize the shrinkage that occurs as kinky-curly hair dries, twist or plait each section and let it air dry.

As mentioned before, Wash & Gos don't work for my type of 4c/4b hair; it shrinks so much that by day 2 styling is too difficult.

When it was shorter I only did 3-strand plaits because they were the most effective at stretching. Now that I have gone past shoulder-length, twisting is faster and it stretches the hair well enough to do all the styles I like.

Finally, to stimulate hair growth I usually finish the wash process by massaging the scalp using *Neno Natural's Hair Growth Stimulator*.

This is just one routine. Your hair management techniques will change with the seasons and with your hair length. Nothing is fixed.

Watch **"The wash-condition-detangle routine that brought my natural African hair back from hell to healthy"** for the routine I used when I first "returned" natural. (youtube.com/watch?v=cjIPu1lnFA0).

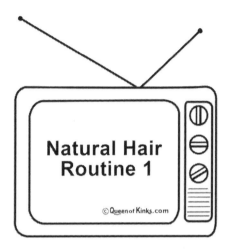

REGIMEN TIP 2: Maintain a daily hair routine whether or not your hair is in braids

Daily Routine For Loose Hair (Not In Braids)

STEP 1: Spritz some water on your twisted or untwisted hair.

If you plan on wearing a protective style you can use as much water as you like. But if you'll be wearing your hair out, use very little water to prevent shrinkage and frizzing.

STEP 2: Cover your head in a shower cap whilst you get ready for the day if your hair is matted or very dry.

STEP 3: Add a little creamy moisturizer, e.g. *Queen of Kinks* 'Protect Me Jealously!'

Moisturizer to soften hair, oil to seal, then style.

STEP 5: Twist your hair before bed, massage an oil plus essential oil blend, e.g. *Neno Natural's Hair Growth Stimulator* into the scalp.

If you don't want to moisturize your entire head of hair, perhaps because you think it'll look too greasy, then only moisturize the ends for hydration.

Daily Routine For Braided Hair

If your hair is in plaits massage an oil such as *Neno Natural's Hair Growth Stimulator* into the scalp daily, especially in the early days to ensure your hair is still in great condition when you unbraid it.

REGIMEN TIP 3: Learn from other people but don't just copy them – adapt their methods to suit your hair

Other People's Regimens

It's all well and good knowing what my regimen is to inform your own; however, I realized that it's useful for everyone to share and learn from each other.

In Dec-2013 I introduced a feature section called the Queen of Kinks, Curls & Coils at NenoNatural.com/queens.

On this section of the website you can learn about other people's regimens (people of different hair types and from different parts of the world) including their top tips and hair tragedies.

You can also email us to be considered for the feature.

At the time of going to press (Sep-2015) over 200 people have been featured at NenoNatural.com/queens.

Chapter 20: Products

PRODUCT TIP 1: Buy the best quality hair care products that you can.

Although it's now relatively easy to find decent products in the US and the UK, there are so many brands to pick from you might need help choosing the best ones.

Every product works for someone, no product works for everyone. Remember, products that work for someone with a similar hair type to you might not work on your hair. You have to go through your own trial and error process.

Mainstream products are cheap because they are mostly **water** and use very few natural ingredients such as butter and oils. The more farm grown ingredients a hair product contains (as opposed to factory chemicals) the more expensive it will be because there is a fixed and limited global supply of them. The plants from which oils and butters are derived only grow in certain climates during specific seasons. Factory ingredients can be created in a factory at any time in any country and are cheaper.

The *Queen of Kinks* product line is designed specifically for dry hair by a top British chemist.

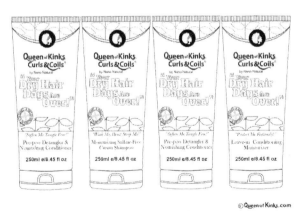

© QueenofKinks.com

To bring a rapid end to dry hair issues get

your product box NOW – the set contains:

- two deep conditioners which also work as pre-shampoo detanglers,
- a super gentle, sulfate-free **cream** shampoo (even the biggest no-poo fan will love it) and
- a leave-in moisturizer.

Your box is waiting for you. Use the coupon code SOFTH4IR on amazon.com or SOFTHAIR on amazon.co.uk and nenonatural.com for a 10% discount. Depending on the length and thickness of your hair a boxed set will last 3 to 6 months. If you have a TWA, it will last longer.

You will find independent reviews on Amazon and on YouTube. You will find YouTubers that have tried the line at NenoNatural.com/queenofkinks.

If you prefer homemade products to commercial ones check out our collection of DIY hair care recipes at NenoNatural.com/courses. When they were launched all our DIY Hair Recipe went to the best seller list and one point all 6 books filled spots 1 to 6 under Best Sellers in Crafts & Hobbies. For more, see: nenonatural.com/hair-blog/diy-hair-product-series-on-promotion-in-kindle-store.

If you try any of our products email the link to your Amazon review to info@nenonatural.com and you will automatically be added to our annual product giveaway in November. We hold a huge giveaway every November.

~ The End ~

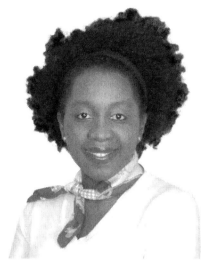

Thank you so much for taking the time to read this book. I would greatly appreciate a book review on Amazon.

For 10% off your order of the *Queen of Kinks* boxed set of products for dry hair, use the coupon code SOFTH4IR on amazon.com or SOFTHAIR on amazon.co.uk and at NenoNatural.com. Quick links are at NenoNatural.com/queenofkinks.

Scan to check out the amazing *Queen of Kinks* product box for dry hair.

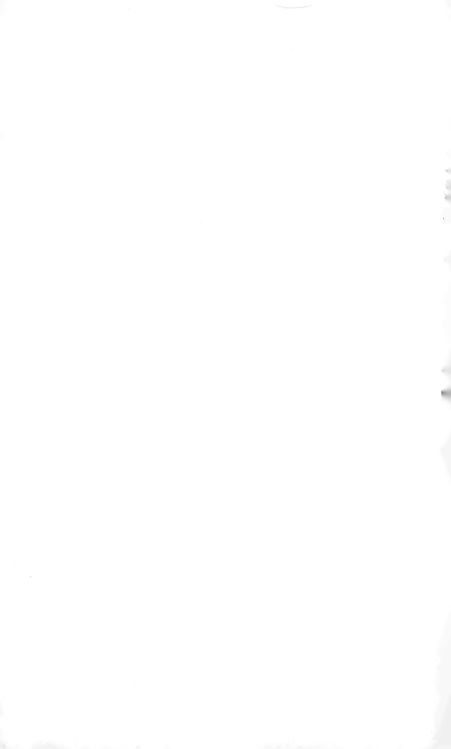